PROMOTING WELLNESS AND PARTICIPATION

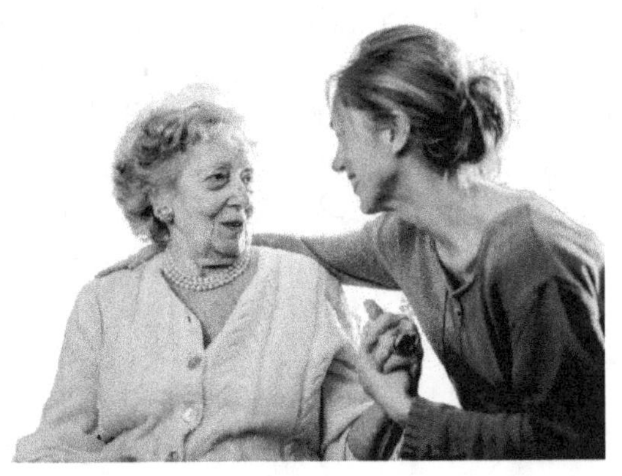

A GUIDE TO LIVING WELL WITH PARKINSON'S DISEASE

Angela K. Butler

DISCLAIMER:

The information contained in this book is for informational purposes only and is not intended to be a substitute for professional advice. While every effort has been made to ensure the accuracy of the information presented, Angela K. Butler and the publisher assume no responsibility for errors or omissions, or for the results obtained from the use of this information. Readers are encouraged to seek professional guidance for their specific needs.

ABOUT THE AUTHOR

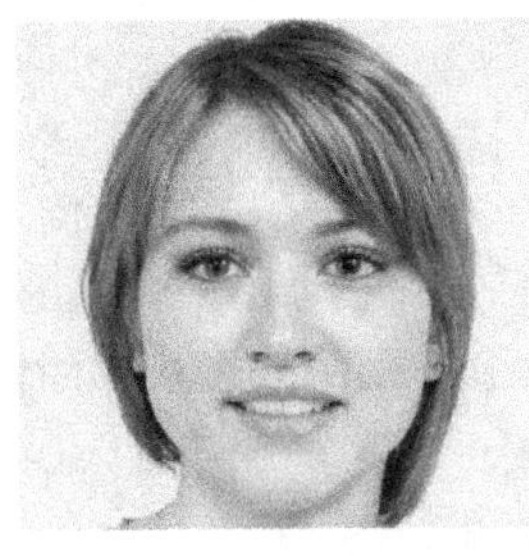 Angela K. Butler is a dedicated occupational therapist who has dedicated her career to empowering individuals living with dementia and their caregivers. With a deep understanding of the cognitive and physical challenges associated with dementia, Angela utilizes her expertise to help people navigate this journey with compassion and knowledge.

Through her work as an occupational therapist, Angela has gained invaluable experience in creating strategies and interventions that promote independence and improve the quality of life for those living with dementia. Her passion lies in empowering individuals to maintain a sense of control and purpose amidst the changing landscape of their cognitive abilities.

Angela's commitment extends beyond the confines of treatment sessions. She is a firm believer in sharing knowledge and resources with the wider community. This captivating book is a testament to that belief.

By offering clear, practical guidance, Angela seeks to equip caregivers and families with the tools they need to provide optimal support for their loved ones.

Driven by a genuine empathy for those affected by dementia, Angela's approach is not only professional but also deeply personal. She understands the emotional complexities that dementia presents, and her writing is infused with a comforting understanding that resonates with readers.

So, whether you are a caregiver seeking practical advice or a loved one looking to gain a better understanding of dementia, Angela K. Butler's book offers a beacon of hope and guidance. Her expertise and genuine care for those living with dementia make her a trusted resource on this often-challenging path.

TABLE OF CONTENT

CHAPTER 1: INTRODUCTION

1.1 Getting to Know Parkinson's Disease

Imagine you're in your favorite dance studio, moving to the music effortlessly. But suddenly, something feels off. Your hand starts shaking, and your steps become unsteady. This is what it's like for many people with Parkinson's disease. It messes up how you move.

Martha, a retired teacher who loves salsa dancing, first noticed a slight shake in her right hand. It started small but got worse over time, making simple tasks like buttoning her shirt hard.
John, on the other hand, was a lifelong athlete. He began feeling stiff in his legs, making it tough to run like he used to. When the doctor said he had Parkinson's, he felt scared.

Parkinson's disease can feel like an unwelcome guest crashing your party, making it hard to enjoy life. It's a brain problem that messes with how you move, causing shaking, stiffness, slowness, and balance issues.

But there's hope. Martha, John, and many others have found ways to live well despite Parkinson's.

This book is your guide to living your best life with Parkinson's. We'll talk about what Parkinson's is, how it affects your daily life, and most importantly, how you can stay healthy and active.

Some people think Parkinson's means your life will only get worse. But that's not true. With the right approach, you can feel better and keep doing what you love. This book will give you practical tips for managing symptoms, staying positive, and staying connected to the things you enjoy.

We'll talk about the science of Parkinson's, but we'll focus on helping you feel empowered. You'll hear from people who have faced Parkinson's and found ways to live well. You'll learn:
- What Parkinson's symptoms are and how they affect your life.
- Why staying active and positive is so important.
- Tips for dealing with shaking, stiffness, and trouble balancing.
- How to handle problems like feeling tired, trouble sleeping, and pain.
- Why setting goals and having support from others is key.

Parkinson's might change how you move, but it doesn't have to stop the music. With the tips in this book, you can find new ways to enjoy life and stay active.

1.2: Understanding Parkinson's Disease

Picture your brain as a big dance studio. Billions of nerve cells work together to make your movements smooth and coordinated. They use certain molecules to communicate with one other. One of these chemicals is called dopamine, and it helps your brain tell your body when to move.

In Parkinson's disease, something goes wrong in this dance studio. The nerve cells that make dopamine start to break down and die. This makes it hard for your brain to control your movements.

Here's what's happening inside your brain:
Dopamine: This chemical tells your brain how to move your muscles smoothly.
Substantia Nigra: It's a small part of your brain that makes dopamine. In Parkinson's, these cells get damaged or die.
Basal Ganglia: This part of your brain helps control your movements. It uses dopamine to tell

your muscles what to do. When there's not enough dopamine, your movements get messed up.

Parkinson's symptoms can be different for everyone, but some common ones include shaking, stiffness, slowness, and trouble balancing.

Remember, Parkinson's affects everyone differently. Some people get worse slowly, while others get worse faster. But there are treatments that can help you feel better and live well with Parkinson's.

Next, we'll talk about how Parkinson's might affect your daily life and what you can do to stay independent and healthy.

1.3: How Parkinson's Disease Affects Your Daily Life

Parkinson's disease can change many parts of your everyday routine, from getting dressed in the morning to doing the things you love. The shaking, stiffness, and slow movements can make even simple tasks feel tough. But the main thing to remember is, with a few changes and a positive mindset, you can adjust your daily life and keep living a satisfying life.

Let's look at some common areas where Parkinson's might make a difference:

- Morning Routine: Stiff muscles can make getting up and getting dressed slow and hard. Think about wearing clothes with buttons or elastic bands. If reaching for things is tough, try moving stuff lower or using tools to grab them.
- Mealtimes: Shaky hands can make holding utensils or eating tricky. Consider using heavier utensils or ones with bigger handles. And using plates with edges can help stop spills.
- Personal Care: Things like showering or shaving might get tricky because of shakes and balance problems. Putting grab bars in the bathroom and using a shower seat can help you stay safe. And electric razors might be easier than manual ones.
- Getting Around: Stiffness and slowness can make walking harder. A physical therapist can teach you exercises to improve your balance and walking. And using a cane or walker for support can make things easier.
- Talking: Moving slowly can sometimes affect your speech. Take your time when you talk and try to speak clearly.

- Feeling Emotions: Getting diagnosed with Parkinson's can be a lot to handle and might make you feel anxious or sad.
  But you're not alone. There are people and groups out there to help you cope with your feelings.

Everyone's experience with Parkinson's is different. The key is to notice where you need help and find ways to make life easier and happier.

Here are some extra tips for dealing with Parkinson's in your daily life:

1. **Plan Ahead:** Do important stuff when you have the most energy. Break big tasks into smaller ones.
2. **Stay Organized:** Keep things you use a lot close by and have a place for everything so you don't waste time looking for stuff.
3. **Ask for Help:** Don't be afraid to get help from family, friends, or caregivers when you need it.
4. **Focus on What You Can Do:** Instead of worrying about what you can't do, focus on the things you can still enjoy and celebrate your victories, no matter how small.

With a positive attitude and a problem-solving mindset, you can make Parkinson's less of a challenge and keep living a meaningful life.

CHAPTER 2: WHY WELLNESS AND BEING INVOLVED MATTER

Imagine you're back in that dance studio we talked about before. The music starts, but this time, things feel heavy and sad. The dancers, representing different parts of your life with Parkinson's – like moving, feeling, and being social – seem stuck, not sure what to do next. It feels like there's no hope.

Then, a spotlight shines on you, but a different you. You're determined, with a spark of hope in your eyes. You take a step, then another, following the music. Slowly, the other dancers start moving too. Their stiffness fades, and they start smiling. The sadness turns into a strong desire to take back control.

That's the power of wellness and being involved. It's about knowing that even though Parkinson's might change how you move, you can still control how you feel. By taking care of yourself and staying active, you can help yourself feel better and deal with challenges.

Wellness: Keeping Everything in Tune:
Think of your well-being like a beautiful song. Each part of your health – like staying active, feeling

good, being social, and taking care of yourself – is like an instrument in an orchestra. When they all work well together, they create a strong and happy tune that helps you live a good life with Parkinson's.

- **Staying Active:** Moving your body helps you stay strong and flexible, like making sure the drums sound good in the orchestra.
- **Feeling Good:** Managing stress and feeling positive helps you deal with problems better, like making sure the violins play the right notes.
- **Being Social:** Connecting with others gives you support and makes you feel like you belong, like the deep sounds of a cello.
- **Taking Care:** Eating well, sleeping enough, and managing medicines keeps you healthy, like making sure all the instruments are in good shape.

Being Involved: Taking the Lead:
Now, think about being involved. This means doing things you enjoy, like hobbies or spending time with friends. It's about being in charge of your life and not letting Parkinson's decide what you can or can't do.

Being involved is important because:

1. Keeps You Going: Doing stuff you like makes you feel good and gives you energy to keep going.
2. Helps Your Brain: Being social and staying busy can slow down Parkinson's.
3. Fights Feeling Alone: Being with others makes you feel like you're part of something and stops you from feeling lonely.
4. Gives You a Reason: Doing stuff you care about gives your life meaning and makes you feel important.

By focusing on wellness and being involved, you're not just dealing with Parkinson's; you're making your life better and happier. You're in control, deciding how you want to live and enjoying every moment.

In the next chapters, we'll talk more about each part of wellness, giving you tips to feel better physically and emotionally, make friends, and stay healthy. We'll also talk about different things you can do to enjoy life and feel like you're in charge, even with Parkinson's.

2.1: How Exercise Helps Your Body

Parkinson's might make it harder to move, but you can still take charge of your physical health. Regular exercise is really important for managing your symptoms and feeling better overall. Here's why:

1. Moving Better: Exercise helps fight the stiffness and slowness that come with Parkinson's. Things like walking, dancing, tai chi, and physical therapy can make it easier to do everyday stuff like getting dressed or walking around the house.

2. Calmer Tremors: Exercise won't make tremors go away completely, but it can make them less intense and happen less often. Doing activities that focus on moving smoothly can really help.

3. Getting Stronger: Regular exercise builds up your muscles, which is super important for staying balanced and doing daily tasks. It also helps you have more energy to do things for longer.

4. Less Risk of Falling: Falls are a big worry for people with Parkinson's because of balance problems. But doing exercises that help you

balance and strengthen your core muscles can make falls less likely.

5. Stronger Bones: Parkinson's can make your bones weaker, but doing exercises like walking or dancing can keep them strong and lower your chances of breaking them.

6. Better Sleep: Exercise can help you fall asleep quicker, sleep better, and feel more rested when you wake up. This is really important because good sleep helps manage Parkinson's symptoms.

7. Sharper Thinking: Regular exercise might slow down the thinking problems that can come with Parkinson's. It can make your memory and focus better.

8. Feeling Good: Exercise is known to boost your mood. It can help you feel less stressed, anxious, or sad – all things that are common with Parkinson's. It also makes you feel happier and offers you more energy.

Remember:
- You can start exercising at any time, even if you've never done it before.
- Check with your doctor first, especially if you have health issues.

- There are lots of exercises that are good for Parkinson's. Find ones you like and can keep doing.
- Doing exercise regularly is important. Try to do at least 30 minutes most days.

2.2: How Being Involved Helps You Feel Better

Parkinson's can make you feel alone and keep you from doing things you enjoy. But being social is really important for feeling good. Here's how being active can help you feel better:

- **Not Feeling Alone:** Being with others makes you feel like you belong and stops you from feeling lonely. Doing things you like with people who understand what you're going through can help you make new friends and share experiences.

- **Feeling Happier:** Being around others makes you feel good and stops you from feeling sad, which can happen with Parkinson's. Hanging out with people gives you a sense of belonging and support. Having a laugh, sharing stories, and chatting with friends can really cheer you up.

- **Thinking Better:** Being social keeps your brain active and helps you stay sharp. Talking to people, doing things in groups, and learning new stuff can all help you think better and slow down thinking problems that come with Parkinson's.

- **Feeling Confident:** Doing things and reaching goals, even small ones, can make you feel good about yourself. It shows you can do stuff and makes you feel proud.

- **Stress Relief:** Talking to others who know what you're going through can help you feel better and learn new ways to cope. Having people who support you can also help you manage stress and worry, which can make Parkinson's symptoms worse.

- **Finding Meaning:** Doing things that matter to you gives your life a sense of purpose. Whether it's helping out, doing stuff you like, or spending time with family, being involved lets you make a difference and feel good about yourself.

1. **Join a Group:** Being with others who understand can really help.
   Support groups are places where you can talk, ask questions, and support each other.
2. **Keep in Touch:** Stay close to family and old friends. Let them know you appreciate them.
3. **Try New Stuff:** Keep learning and trying new things. Find things you enjoy, like a book club, walking group, or art class.
4. **Help Out:** Giving back to your community feels good and keeps you busy.
5. **Use Technology:** Keep in touch with faraway friends and family with video calls or social media. Online groups for people with Parkinson's can also be helpful.

Even small steps can make a big difference. Don't be scared to try new things and connect with others. Being involved will help you feel better, find support, and enjoy spending time with people.

CHAPTER 3: EXERCISE FOR FEELING GOOD

Dealing with Parkinson's can make moving harder, but it doesn't mean you can't stay active. In fact, exercise is a great way to manage your symptoms, feel better overall, and live a satisfying life. This chapter will help you discover different exercises that suit your needs, so you can move confidently and enjoyably.

Why Exercise Is Awesome:

Let's remind ourselves of the amazing benefits exercise brings for people with Parkinson's:

Better Moving: Exercise fights stiffness and slowness, making it easier to do everyday tasks and reducing your chances of falling.

Calmer Tremors: While it won't stop tremors completely, exercise can make them less intense and happen less often.

Stronger and More Energy: Regular exercise builds muscles and helps you have more stamina for activities.

Sleeping Better: Exercise helps you sleep deeper and feel more awake during the day.

Sharper Thinking: Keeping active helps your brain stay sharp and can slow down thinking problems.

Feeling Happier: Exercise boosts your mood and reduces stress, anxiety, and depression.

Picking the Right Exercise for You:

To make your exercise routine work, consider these things:

Start Where You're At: Begin with exercises that match your abilities and work your way up.

Think About Your Symptoms: Choose exercises that help with your specific symptoms, like balance or stiffness.

Do What You Like: Pick activities that you enjoy – it'll make sticking to them easier.

Make It Doable: Check if the exercise is accessible in terms of location, equipment, and cost.

Great Exercises to Try:

Gentle Activities:

- Walking: Start with short walks and gradually increase the time and distance.
- Swimming: Enjoy a full-body workout with the support of water.
- Yoga: Gentle poses improve flexibility, balance, and core strength.
- Tai Chi: Combines movement, breathing, and meditation to boost balance and well-being.

Medium-Intensity Moves:

- Dancing: Choose a style you like to improve coordination and flexibility.
- Cycling: Whether indoors or outdoors, it's a great way to exercise your legs and core.
- Circuit Training: Switch between exercises to work different muscle groups.

Building Strength:
- Light Weights: Start with light weights to improve muscle mass and balance.
- Resistance Bands: Versatile bands help build strength safely at home.

Tips for a Successful Workout:
1. Warm Up and Cool Down:* Start with a gentle warm-up and end with a cool-down to prevent injuries and soreness.
2. Listen to Your Body: Don't overdo it – take breaks and gradually increase intensity.
3. Stay Hydrated: Drink plenty of water before, during, and after exercise.
4. Talk to a Pro: Discuss your plans with your doctor or physical therapist to make sure they're safe for you.

Don't worry about the limitations – there's an exercise out there for everyone. Just find what works for you and enjoy the benefits of staying active with Parkinson's.

3.1: Easy Exercises and Physical Therapy - Building Your Strength

Dealing with Parkinson's can make simple tasks tough, but starting with gentle exercises and working with a physical therapist can really help. These approaches lay a strong foundation for improving your movement, balance, and overall well-being.

The Magic of Gentle Exercise:
Regular easy exercises offer many benefits for people with Parkinson's disease:
Getting More Flexible: Gentle stretches loosen tight muscles and let you move more freely. This makes daily activities like reaching or dressing up easier.
Imagine stretching your arms out to grab something high up. If your shoulders feel stiff, gentle arm stretches can make reaching easier.

Getting Steadier on Your Feet: Exercises focusing on shifting your weight or standing on one leg can really improve your balance. This lowers your risk of falls, which is a big worry for people with Parkinson's.

Think of yourself balancing on a beam. Exercises can help you stay steady and centered, just like a skilled acrobat.

Calming the Tremors: Doing gentle, rhythmic movements like walking or swinging your arms can lessen the shakiness.
Imagine holding a cup of coffee. If tremors make it wobble, gentle arm exercises can help steady your hands.

Getting Stronger: Even light exercises can help you keep muscles strong, which is important for supporting your body and moving better.
Imagine climbing stairs. Stronger legs make each step more stable and confident.

Examples of Easy Exercises:
Here are some simple exercises you can easily add to your routine:
- Walking: Start with short walks and gradually go longer as you get stronger.
- Stretching: Gentle stretches for your arms, legs, neck, and back can help with flexibility and stiffness.
- Heel-Toe Walking: Walk by placing your heel in front of your toe with each step. This helps with balance and coordination.
- Arm Circles: Make small circles with your arms forward and backward.

- This loosens your shoulders and makes your upper body more flexible.
- Tai Chi: This slow, graceful practice with deep breathing helps with balance, coordination, and relaxation.

Physical Therapy: Your Personal Movement Guide

A physical therapist (PT) knows a lot about movement problems and can make a special exercise plan just for you. Here's how a PT can help:

- Finding What You Need: A PT will check how strong, flexible, balanced, and how you walk you are. Then they'll make a plan to help you.
- Making Your Own Plan: Your PT will make an exercise plan just for you that helps you reach your goals.
- Teaching You the Right Way: Your PT will show you how to do the exercises the right way so you stay safe and get the most benefit.
- Cheering You On: Your PT can help you stay motivated and support you as you work on your exercises.

More Good Stuff About Physical Therapy:

Stopping Falls: PTs can teach you exercises and tricks to help you keep your balance and not fall.

Less Pain: Exercises from a PT can help you deal with any pain you have from Parkinson's.

CHAPTER 4: TAKING CARE OF YOUR FEELING

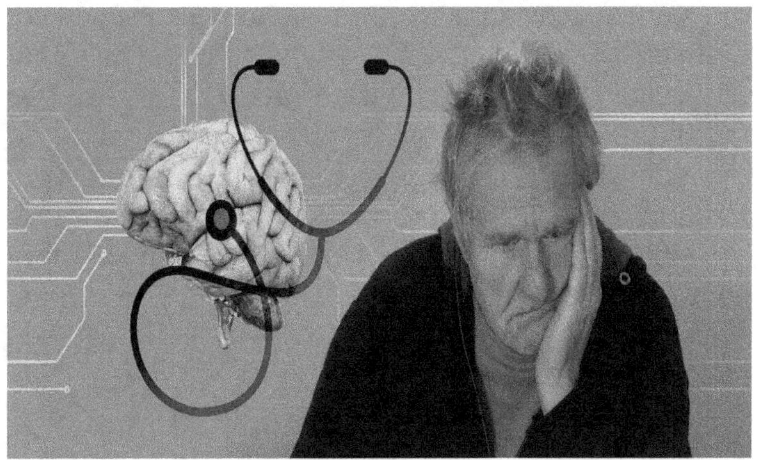

Parkinson's disease can bring up a lot of different feelings. The diagnosis alone can be a lot to handle, and dealing with the physical challenges can leave you feeling frustrated, worried, or down. But here's some good news: you're not alone in this. By making your emotional well-being a priority, you can find strength within yourself, handle tough emotions, and still lead a fulfilling life despite Parkinson's.

Understanding How You Feel:

Parkinson's can mess with both your body and your emotions. These are some emotions that you may feel.:

Feeling Down: You might feel sad, lose interest in things you used to enjoy, or just feel really down.

Feeling Anxious: Worries about the future, managing your symptoms, or losing your independence can make you feel anxious and scared.

Getting Frustrated: The slow movements and stiffness that come with Parkinson's can be frustrating, especially when you're just trying to do everyday stuff.

Feeling Angry: Feeling stuck or powerless because of your limitations might make you feel angry sometimes.

Grieving: It's okay to feel sad about the things you can't do anymore and the life you had before.

Ways to Take Care of Your Emotions:
Even though Parkinson's can make you feel these things, you don't have to let it control you. Here are some ways to take care of your emotions:

1. Let Yourself Feel:** It's okay to feel sad, mad, or frustrated. Talk about how you're feeling with someone you trust, like a friend, family member, or therapist.
2. Fight Negative Thoughts: Parkinson's might make you think bad stuff about yourself. Challenge those thoughts. Focus on what you

can do and be proud of your accomplishments, no matter how small.

3. Relax Your Mind: Stuff like deep breathing, meditation, or just chilling out can help you deal with stress and anxiety.
4. Stay Positive: Think about the things you're thankful for and the good stuff in your life. Seek for the things that provide you joy and purpose in life.
5. Ask for Help: If you're feeling really down or anxious, don't be afraid to talk to a therapist or counselor. They can help you figure things out and support you.

Taking Care of Yourself:

Looking after your emotional well-being also means taking care of yourself. The following are some helpful things:

- Get Good Sleep: Sleep is super important for your body and mind. Try to get 7-8 hours of good sleep every night.
- Eat Healthy: Good food gives your brain and body the stuff they need to handle stress and stay balanced.
- Drink Water: Staying hydrated keeps you feeling good and helps your body work right.
- Hang Out with Loved Ones: Spending time with friends and family who get what you're going through can make a big difference.

Accepting Where You're At:

Parkinson's is something you'll have for a while, so there might be times when you feel down. But it's important to accept it and keep going. Here's how:

- Focus on What You Can Do: Don't dwell on what you can't do anymore. Focus on what you still can do and find ways to adjust and stay independent.
- Celebrate Little Wins: Every win, no matter how small, is a big deal. Be proud of what you've accomplished and how strong you are.
- Live for Today: Don't worry too much about the past or the future. Enjoy what's happening right now and make the most of each day.
- Find Meaning: Doing stuff that matters to you, like helping others, doing hobbies, or spending time with loved ones, can make you feel better.

Taking care of your emotions is a journey. There'll be good days and tough ones, but by looking after yourself, asking for help when you need it, and accepting where you're at, you can find strength and handle the emotions that come with Parkinson's.

4.1: Handling Stress and Anxiety

Dealing with Parkinson's disease can bring a lot of stress and worry. Just knowing you have it and managing the symptoms can make you feel overwhelmed. But here's something empowering: you've got what it takes to handle these feelings and find peace within yourself.

Understanding Stress and Anxiety:
Feeling stressed or anxious is normal when you're facing tough situations. Whether it's worrying about what's ahead, managing your health, or keeping your independence, it's natural to feel this way. But if stress and anxiety stick around too long, they can make things harder, including your Parkinson's symptoms.

How Stress and Anxiety Affect Parkinson's:

Here's how ongoing stress and anxiety can show up when you have Parkinson's:
- Making Tremors Worse: Stress can make your tremors more noticeable and harder to control.
- Tensing Up Muscles: Anxiety can make your muscles tight, making it harder to move comfortably.
- Messing with Sleep: Stress and anxiety can mess up your sleep, making it tough to fall asleep or stay asleep. This can leave you feeling tired and make your symptoms feel worse.

- Trouble Focusing: Anxiety can make it hard to concentrate, making everyday tasks more challenging.
- Feeling Less Motivated: When stress and anxiety pile up, it can be tough to feel motivated to do things you used to enjoy.

Ways to Deal with Stress and Anxiety:

Luckily, there are ways to handle stress and anxiety and feel more in control of your emotions:

1. Figure Out What's Stressing You: First, figure out what's making you feel stressed or anxious. Is it worrying about your symptoms, what's ahead, or just feeling overwhelmed?
2. Challenge Negative Thoughts: Stress often makes you think bad stuff about yourself. Challenge those thoughts and focus on the good things you can do and how strong you are.
3. Relax Your Mind: Things like deep breathing, muscle relaxation, and meditation can really help calm you down.

Here's a simple deep breathing exercise you can try:
- Look for a peaceful area where you won't be bothered.
- Sit or lie down comfortably and close your eyes.

- Breathe in slowly and deeply through your nose for a count of four.
- Hold your breath for two counts.
- Breathe out slowly through your mouth for a count of six.
- Repeat this for 5-10 minutes.

4. Remain Upbeat: Pay attention to the positive aspects of your life. Be thankful for what you have and celebrate your victories, no matter how small.

5. Keep Moving: Regular exercise is a great way to bust stress. Whether it's walking, swimming, or yoga, staying active can really help you feel better. Check out Chapter 3 for exercise ideas.

6. Talk to Someone: Having people you can talk to and lean on is important. Talk to a therapist, family member, or trusted friend about your concerns.

7. Mindfulness Meditation: This kind of meditation helps you focus on the present and accept your thoughts and feelings without judging them. It's a great way to ease stress and anxiety.

Cognitive Behavioral Therapy (CBT):
If stress and anxiety are really getting in the way of your daily life, think about seeing a therapist who knows about Cognitive Behavioral Therapy (CBT).

It's a kind of therapy that teaches you how to deal with negative thoughts that make you stressed and anxious.

Living with Less Stress:
Dealing with stress and anxiety is an ongoing thing. Here are some more tips for keeping stress in check:

- Set Small Goals: Break big tasks into smaller ones. It'll make you feel more accomplished and less overwhelmed.
- Learn to Say No: Don't feel bad about turning down stuff that'll stress you out. Put your well-being first.
- Ask for Help: You don't have to do everything yourself. Ask friends, family, or pros for help when you need it.
- Manage Your Time: Good time management can keep you from feeling rushed and stressed.
- Find Joy: Laughter is a great way to bust stress. Do things that make you happy and laugh often.

By dealing with stress and anxiety head-on, you'll create a calmer inner space and feel stronger emotionally as you handle life with Parkinson's. Next up, we'll talk about why getting enough good sleep matters and how it can make a big difference in how you feel overall.

4.2: Strengthening Your Inner Strength and Positive Coping

Facing Parkinson's disease can bring unexpected hurdles, but you're not alone in overcoming them. Building inner strength – the ability to bounce back from tough times – is crucial for handling the ups and downs of this condition. This section gives you practical ways to tackle obstacles, deal with setbacks, and lead a fulfilling life despite the challenges of Parkinson's.

Why Building Inner Strength Matters:
Living with Parkinson's disease means facing both triumphs and trials. Strengthening your inner resilience helps you:

Adapt to Change: Parkinson's is progressive, meaning symptoms might worsen over time. Inner strength helps you adjust to these changes and stay in control of your life.

Handle Setbacks: Everyone faces setbacks. Inner strength gives you the tools to bounce back from tough days, medication effects, or unexpected issues.

Keep a Positive Outlook: Having a positive mindset doesn't mean ignoring difficulties. Inner strength helps you find hope and positivity, even in tough times.

Live a Meaningful Life: Building inner strength lets you focus on what you can control and find ways to enjoy life despite Parkinson's.

Developing Healthy Coping Strategies:
Coping strategies are your tools for managing stress, anxiety, and emotional challenges linked to Parkinson's. The following are some useful tactics to cultivate:

- Problem-Solving: Face challenges head-on by identifying problems, brainstorming solutions, and choosing the best path forward.
- Positive Thinking: Replace negative thoughts with positive ones. Focus on your strengths and past successes. Tell yourself, "I can handle this" or "I've overcome obstacles before, and I can do it again."
- Acceptance: Understand that Parkinson's is part of your life, but it doesn't define it. Concentrate on what you can control and make each day count.
- Gratitude: Being thankful for the good things, no matter how small, can boost your mood and resilience.
- Humor: Find the funny side of life's situations. Laughter is a great way to relieve stress and lighten your mood.

Building Your Support Network:
These are some emotions that you may feel. Here's how to build yours:
1. Connect with Loved Ones: Spend time with understanding family and friends who can offer support and encouragement.
2. Join Support Groups: Being around others who understand Parkinson's can be invaluable. Support groups provide a safe space to share experiences and get encouragement.
3. Seek Professional Help: Don't hesitate to reach out to a therapist if you're struggling with stress, anxiety, or other emotional challenges. They can offer assistance and coping mechanisms.

More Ways to Boost Resilience:
1. Healthy Living: Prioritize sleep, nutrition, and exercise to enhance your overall well-being and resilience.
2. Meaningful Activities: Engage in hobbies or volunteer work that brings you joy and purpose. Adapt activities to fit your abilities.
3. Celebrate Wins: Acknowledge and celebrate even small achievements. It strengthens your sense of accomplishment.

4. Be Present: Focus on the here and now instead of dwelling on the past or worrying about the future. Practice mindfulness to enjoy each moment fully.

Building inner strength is an ongoing journey. There will be good days and tough days, but by focusing on your strengths and celebrating victories, you'll discover just how resilient you truly are.

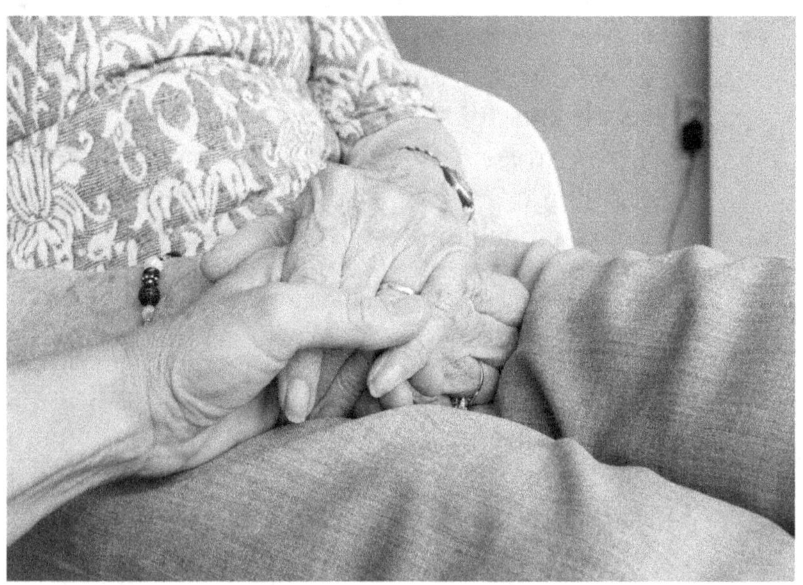

CHAPTER 5: SOCIAL CONNECTION AND BEING ACTIVE

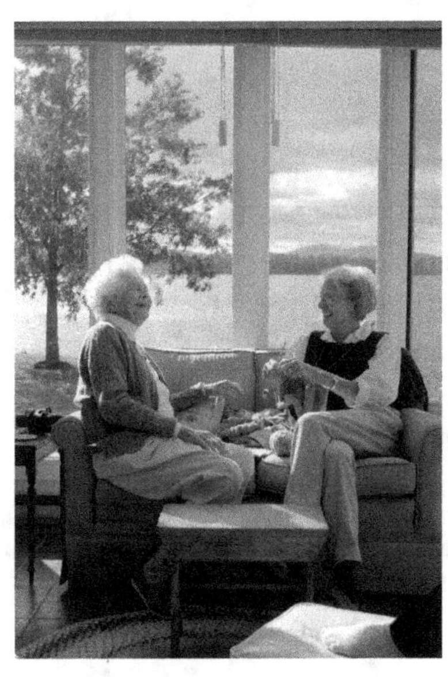

Parkinson's disease might sometimes make you feel alone. Its physical and emotional challenges might tempt you to avoid socializing. But here's something important: staying connected with others and staying involved in life are crucial for your well-being. This chapter explains why social interaction matters and gives tips on staying connected and finding purpose despite Parkinson's.

The Importance of Being Social:
Humans naturally need social interaction. It's vital for emotional well-being and overall health, especially with Parkinson's disease:
- **Fighting Loneliness:** Being with others reduces feelings of loneliness and isolation.

Doing activities you enjoy lets you make friends and share experiences with people who understand what you're going through.

- **Improving Mood:** Socializing boosts positive feelings and fights depression, common in Parkinson's. Laughing, talking, and connecting with others lifts your spirits.
- **Keeping Sharp:** Interacting with others stimulates your brain and keeps your mind active.
Chatting, doing group activities, and learning new things help keep your brain in shape.
- Boosting Confidence: Being active and achieving goals, no matter how small, boosts your confidence and self-esteem.

Benefits of Staying Active:

Being active isn't just about socializing; it's about doing things that make you happy and fulfilled:

1. Less Stress: Sharing your experiences with others reduces stress and gives you helpful coping strategies.
2. Finding Purpose: Doing meaningful activities gives your life direction and meaning, whether it's volunteering or spending time with loved ones.

Staying Connected and Active:
Here's how to stay connected and involved:
Join Support Groups: Connecting with others who understand Parkinson's is helpful. Support groups give you a safe place to share and get support.
Reach Out to Loved Ones: Keep in touch with family and friends. Tell them how much you value their assistance.
Try New Things: Explore hobbies and interests. Keep learning and trying new activities.
Volunteer: Giving back to your community is rewarding and keeps you active.
Use Technology: Stay in touch with distant loved ones through video calls or social media.

Making It Work for You:
Parkinson's might require adjustments, but you can still stay active:

1. Plan Ahead: Consider your energy levels and medication schedule when planning activities.
2. Break Tasks Down: Large tasks can be overwhelming. Break them into smaller steps.
3. Ask for Help: Don't hesitate to ask friends, family, or caregivers for assistance.
4. Focus on Enjoyment: It's okay not to be perfect. Focus on enjoying yourself and the company of others.

 Many resources and support systems are available to help you stay connected and active despite Parkinson's. By following these tips and seeking help when needed, you can continue living a fulfilling life, despite the challenges.

5.1: The Value of Social Bonds - Breaking Barriers, Building Bridges

Living with Parkinson's disease can make you feel like you're losing touch with the world around you. It might seem like the condition steals your ability to connect with others, leaving you feeling isolated. However, maintaining strong social connections is essential for your well-being, and there are ways to nurture them despite the hurdles.

Why Social Connection Is Important:
Humans thrive on connection. Having strong social bonds isn't just nice to have; it's crucial for your mental and physical health. Here's why staying socially engaged matters when you have Parkinson's:

Overcoming Isolation: Loneliness can take a toll on your emotional health. Social interaction bridges the gap, making you feel less alone. Forming friendships and sharing experiences with empathetic individuals who understand your journey can be incredibly comforting.

Imagine being stranded on an island. Though you have what you need to survive, the isolation eventually wears you down. Social connection acts as a bridge, leading you to a vibrant mainland where support, laughter, and belonging await.

Lifting Spirits: Engaging with others sparks joy, laughter, and shared memories, lifting your mood and easing feelings of depression, often experienced with Parkinson's disease.

Keeping Sharp: Socializing is like a mental workout. Conversations, group activities, and learning new things challenge your brain, helping to maintain cognitive function and mental sharpness.

Think of your brain as a muscle. Social interaction is the exercise that keeps it strong and functioning at its best.

Boosting Confidence: Accomplishing tasks, no matter how small, can boost your confidence and self-esteem. Demonstrating your abilities and experiencing a sense of achievement empowers you and fosters a positive self-image.

Picture yourself climbing a mountain. Reaching the peak, despite the challenges, fills you with pride and bolsters your confidence. Social interaction helps you conquer daily peaks in life.

Benefits Extend Beyond Yourself:
Strong social connections benefit not only you but also those around you. Here's how:

- Easing Caregiver Burdens: Your support network lightens the load for caregivers, offering reassurance that you have others to lean on.
- Strengthening Family Bonds: Staying connected with family members strengthens your relationship and creates lasting memories.
- Raising Awareness: Being open about your condition and engaging in social activities can raise awareness and understanding in your community, fostering inclusivity.

Social connection is a two-way street. By reaching out and connecting with others, you not only enrich your own life but also positively impact those around you.

5.2: Tips for Forming Social Ties

Parkinson's disease can present challenges to socializing, but you can still build strong connections despite these obstacles. Understanding and addressing potential barriers is the first step. Here's how:

Spotting Challenges:

Recognize the hurdles that might hinder your social life:

- Physical Limits: Stiffness, tremors, and fatigue can make certain activities challenging.
- Communication Struggles: Difficulty speaking clearly might affect interactions.
- Fear of Judgment: Concerns about how others perceive your symptoms may lead to isolation.
- Depression and Anxiety: Emotional struggles can dampen motivation for socializing.

Overcoming Obstacles:

Once you've identified barriers, try these strategies:

1. Focus on Abilities: Concentrate on what you can do, not what you can't.
2. Plan Wisely: Schedule outings when you have the most energy and pace yourself.
3. Adapt: Use tools or techniques to manage symptoms, like weighted cups for tremors.
4. Communicate Clearly: Inform others about communication challenges and speak slowly.
5. Challenge Assumptions: Don't assume people will judge you negatively.
6. Seek Support: Professional help can assist with overcoming depression or anxiety.
7. Balance Independence and Help: Maintain independence while accepting assistance when needed.

Nurturing Connections:

Now, actively engage in social activities:

Reach Out: Connect with old friends and family via calls or video chats.

Join Groups: Support groups provide understanding and encouragement.

Try New Things: Explore hobbies suitable for your abilities.

Give Back: Volunteering boosts mood and connects you with others.

Embrace Technology: Stay in touch with loved ones through online platforms.

Social Event Success:

Make the most of social gatherings with these tips:

1. Choose Wisely: Opt for well-lit venues with good sound quality.
2. Prepare: Arrange transportation and bring necessary items.
3. Bring Support: A trusted friend can ease anxiety and assist during events.
4. Manage Expectations: Pace yourself and prioritize meaningful conversations.
5. Quality Over Quantity: Focus on deep connections rather than trying to interact with everyone.

CHAPTER 6: CONQUERING CHALLENGES FOR BETTER LIVING

Parkinson's disease brings various hurdles affecting your physical, emotional, and social aspects of life. Yet, there's hope. By actively addressing these obstacles using the strategies outlined below, you can lead a fulfilling life despite the condition.

Common Obstacles to Well-being and Engagement:
Many facing Parkinson's encounter these challenges:

1. Physical Limitations: Stiffness, tremors, fatigue, and balance issues hamper daily tasks and exercise.
2. Pain Management: Persistent pain disrupts mobility and overall well-being.
3. Cognitive Issues: Memory lapses and difficulty focusing pose hurdles.
4. Emotional Struggles: Depression, anxiety, and frustration are common reactions.
5. Social Isolation: Communication barriers and physical limitations lead to withdrawal.
6. Lack of Knowledge and Support:Access to information and support varies.

Ways to Overcome These Barriers:
Effective strategies help navigate these challenges:
- Collaborate with Healthcare Professionals:A dedicated team can tailor a treatment plan to your needs.
- Prioritize Physical Activity: Even modified exercises enhance mobility and well-being.
- Manage Pain: Discuss pain relief methods with your doctor, such as medication and therapy.
- Seek Emotional Support: Therapy aids in coping with emotional challenges.
- Stay Connected: Maintaining social ties alleviates loneliness and boosts mood.
- Educate Yourself: Knowledge empowers you to make informed decisions about your health.
- Advocate for Yourself: Speak up about your needs and seek assistance when necessary.

The Positive Impact of Overcoming Challenges:
Taking charge of your health can lead to a ripple effect of positivity:

Maria's Journey:
After Maria's Parkinson's diagnosis, she faced initial fear and difficulty. However, she gradually regained strength and confidence through small steps like daily stretches and joining support groups. Her

resilience inspired others and showcased the transformative power of overcoming challenges.

With the right tools, support, and mindset, you can conquer the barriers posed by Parkinson's and live a meaningful and joyful life.

6.1: Battling Fatigue and Sleep Issues - Regaining Vitality Despite Challenges

Fatigue and sleep troubles often accompany Parkinson's disease, draining your energy and disrupting your rest. Yet, there's hope. By understanding these issues and implementing effective strategies, you can boost your energy levels and enhance sleep quality.

Grasping Fatigue and Sleep Challenges:
Fatigue: Unlike regular tiredness, Parkinson's-related fatigue persists despite rest, affecting motivation and overall well-being.
Sleep Problems: Difficulty falling asleep, staying asleep, or waking up unrested are common, stemming from factors like dopamine deficiency, medication side effects, pain, and emotional struggles.

Various factors contribute to these issues:
- Dopamine Deficiency: Parkinson's disrupts dopamine levels, impacting sleep regulation.
- Medications: Some drugs used for Parkinson's treatment can induce drowsiness or insomnia.
- Pain and Stiffness: Chronic discomfort makes it hard to find a comfortable sleeping position.
- Emotional Factors: Depression and anxiety disrupt sleep patterns.
- Apnea: Sleep apnea, common in Parkinson's, interrupts sleep cycles.

Breaking the Cycle:
Fatigue and sleep problems often create a harmful cycle, hindering activity levels and perpetuating poor sleep habits.

Strategies to Break the Cycle:
Combat these issues with effective methods:
- Enhance Sleep Hygiene: Establish a consistent sleep schedule and create a soothing bedtime routine.
- Stay Active: Regular exercise improves sleep quality and boosts energy levels.

- Pain Management: Seek effective pain relief methods from your healthcare provider.
- Address Emotional Challenges:Professional help can alleviate depression and anxiety.
- Medication Adjustments: Consult your doctor for medication adjustments to improve sleep.
- Control Napping: Avoid lengthy naps to prevent nighttime sleep disturbances.
- Watch Caffeine and Alcohol: Limit consumption, especially before bedtime, to avoid interference with sleep.
- Light Exposure: Morning light exposure regulates sleep-wake cycles.
- Relaxation Techniques: Practice relaxation exercises like deep breathing before sleep.

Consult your doctor for tailored advice on managing fatigue and sleep problems. By adopting these strategies and collaborating with your healthcare team, you can break free from the cycle and regain energy for a fulfilling life.

6.2: Coping with Pain and Physical Challenges

Parkinson's disease often brings forth a range of physical hurdles, such as pain, stiffness, tremors, and balance issues, affecting daily life and overall well-being. Yet, with effective pain management and proactive approaches, you can take charge of your comfort and uphold your independence.

Understanding Physical Challenges:
1. Pain: Many with Parkinson's endure persistent pain, stemming from muscle stiffness, joint issues, or medication effects.
2. Stiffness: Rigidity, a common symptom, hinders movement and flexibility.
3. Tremors: Involuntary shaking, prevalent in Parkinson's, affects various body parts.
4. Balance Problems: These raise fall risks, impacting mobility and confidence.

Daily Life Impact:
These challenges alter daily routines in several ways:
Mobility Constraints: Tasks like dressing become arduous due to stiffness and tremors.
Dependency: Relying on aid for tasks affects independence.

Fall Risks: Balance issues lead to injuries and limit activity.

Reduced Participation: Pain and limitations curtail enjoyable activities.

Emotional Strain: Chronic pain and constraints lead to anxiety and depression.

Taking Charge:

Implement strategies to manage challenges and regain comfort:

- Pain Relief: Seek effective strategies like medication or therapy.
- Exercise: Regular routines improve flexibility and reduce stiffness.
- Therapy: Customized programs enhance strength, balance, and coordination.
- Assistive Tools: Devices aid in daily tasks, ensuring safety and independence.
- Temperature Therapy: Heat or cold packs offer temporary relief.
- Relaxation: Techniques like deep breathing ease stress and tension.
- Weight Management: Maintaining a healthy weight reduces strain on joints.
- Posture: Good posture enhances balance and reduces pain.
- Fall Prevention: Consult with doctors to assess and prevent fall risks.

Managing Tremors:

Handle tremors with these strategies:
- Stress Management: Relaxation curbs tremors exacerbated by stress.
- Adapt Tools: Larger handles or weighted utensils ease tasks.
- Medication Review: Discuss adjustments to Parkinson's meds with your doctor.

By implementing these strategies, you can effectively cope with physical challenges and maintain a comfortable and independent lifestyle despite Parkinson's disease.

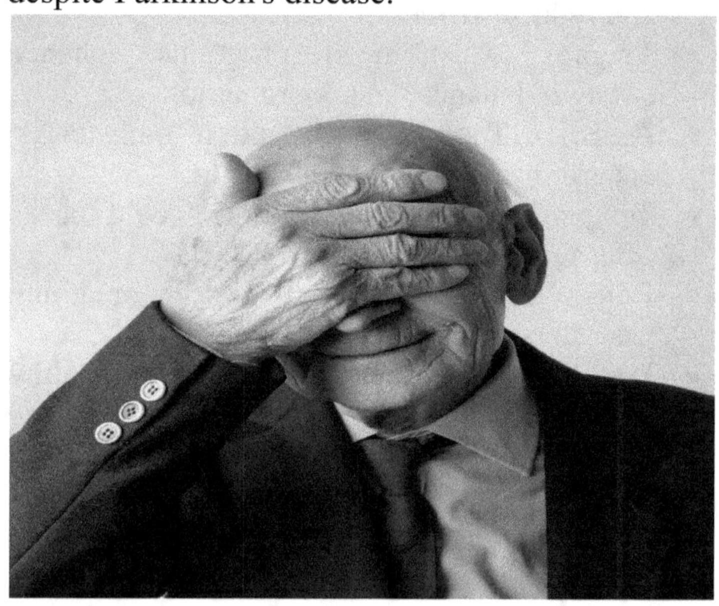

CHAPTER 7: ACHIEVING FEASIBLE OBJECTIVES AND PREFERENCES

Parkinson's disease can disrupt your life and make planning for the future difficult. However, there's an empowering reality: by setting practical goals and effectively prioritizing, you can navigate your journey with Parkinson's disease and attain a satisfying and purposeful life. This chapter equips you with the tools to chart a path toward success, one step at a time.

Importance of Goal Setting:

Establishing goals offers direction, incentive, and a sense of achievement. It enables you to:

1. Maintain Control: Actively setting goals empowers you to manage your health and well-being, rather than letting Parkinson's disease control your life.

2. Boost Motivation: Goals provide a clear target, keeping you motivated and engaged in managing your condition.

3. Celebrate Progress: Achieving goals, regardless of size, is cause for celebration,

reinforcing a sense of accomplishment and propelling you forward.

4. Enhance Overall Well-being: Setting goals encompassing physical activity, healthy eating, social interaction, and emotional well-being contributes to a holistically healthier life with Parkinson's disease.

Significance of Prioritization:

Not all goals carry the same weight. Prioritization helps you focus on the most crucial aspects of your health and well-being. Here's why prioritization is essential:

Limited Energy: Parkinson's disease may limit your energy levels, making it crucial to focus on the most important goals.

Reduced Stress: Prioritization prevents feeling overwhelmed by avoiding taking on too much, reducing stress.

Increased Efficiency: Focusing on priorities allows you to achieve more with the energy you have.

SMART Goal Setting:

When setting goals, remember the SMART criteria:

- Specific: Make goals specific and measurable to provide clear direction, like aiming for "walk for 30 minutes three times a week" instead of the vague "be more active."

- Measurable: Tracking progress with quantifiable measurements or checklists keeps motivation high.
- Attainable: Set challenging yet realistic goals based on your current abilities to avoid discouragement.
- Relevant: Align goals with your values and desires, ensuring they are meaningful and impactful.
- Time-bound: Establish a timeframe for reaching goals to create urgency and maintain focus.

Prioritizing Goals:
After creating a list of SMART goals, prioritize them based on importance and urgency.

Importance: Assess the impact of each goal on your overall well-being, focusing on those that will make the most significant difference.

Urgency: Address goals requiring immediate action first, considering time-sensitive challenges.

Prioritization is an ongoing process; regularly revisit goals and adjust priorities as needed.

Additional tips for successful goal setting and prioritization:

1. Break Down Goals: Divide larger goals into manageable steps to reduce overwhelm.
2. Celebrate Milestones: Acknowledge and celebrate progress to stay motivated along the way.
3. Stay Flexible: Be prepared to adjust goals or priorities in response to changing circumstances.
4. Seek Support: Do not be afraid to seek friends, family, or medical experts for assistance.

Example: Setting a SMART Goal:
Goal: Reduce fall risk by improving balance.

Specific: Attend a balance and gait class twice a week for 12 weeks.

Measurable: Track attendance and improvements in balance tests.

Attainable: Classes are available locally and fit into my schedule.

Relevant: Improving balance enhances safety and enables participation in enjoyable activities.

Time-bound: Complete the 12-week balance and gait class program.

Setting realistic goals and effective prioritization empower you to manage Parkinson's disease and achieve a fulfilling life. Subsequent chapters will explore specific aspects of Parkinson's management, providing the knowledge and tools to create a personalized path to success.

7.1: Grasping the SMART Goals Approach

Parkinson's disease may cast uncertainty on future plans, yet establishing effective goals empowers you to seize control, stay driven, and lead a rewarding life despite the hurdles. This subchapter delves into the SMART Goals methodology, a tool for crafting feasible and impactful goals.

Rationale Behind SMART Goals:
Consider the analogy of scaling a mountain. Ambiguous objectives like "reach the summit" offer little guidance and may lead to confusion or exhaustion. The SMART Goals framework, however, acts as a roadmap, enhancing the likelihood of summiting successfully.

Decoding SMART:
SMART, an acronym, stands for:
- Specific:
- Measurable:
- Attainable:
- Relevant:
- Time-bound:

Let's dissect each aspect and its relevance to goal setting in Parkinson's disease management:

1. Specific:
Ambiguous goals lack clarity and direction. To ensure specificity:

Define the intended outcome: What precisely do you aim to achieve?

Concentrate on one goal at a time: Breaking larger objectives into specific, manageable sub-goals prevents overwhelm.

Example (Ambiguous): "Be more active."

Example (Specific): "Engage in a 30-minute walk, thrice weekly."

2. Measurable:
How will progress be gauged? Measurable goals allow for tracking and motivation:
Quantify objectives: Whenever feasible, employ numerical metrics.
Monitor progress: Utilize journals, checklists, or fitness trackers to track achievements.

Example (Non-Measurable): "Enhance balance."

Example (Measurable): "Decrease sway time in balance tests by 10% within four weeks."

3. Attainable:
Unrealistic goals may lead to discouragement. To ensure attainability:
Assess current capabilities: Set goals challenging yet within reach considering existing limitations.
Commence with modest objectives, escalating gradually: Building skills and confidence starts with manageable steps.
Example (Unrealistic): "Complete a marathon in six months." (For someone lacking recent running experience)
Example (Attainable): "Initiate a beginner's walking regimen, progressively increasing distance weekly."

4. Relevant:
All goals are not created equal. To ensure relevance:

Align goals with personal values and aspirations: What truly matters to you?

Evaluate impact on well-being: How will achieving the goal enhance overall health and quality of life with Parkinson's disease?

Example (Irrelevant): "Master piano playing" (if music holds no interest)

Example (Relevant): "Participate in a Parkinson's-friendly dance class" (enhances balance, coordination, and social engagement)

5. Time-bound:

Timelines instill urgency and focus. To establish time-bound goals:

Set deadlines: When do you intend to achieve the goal? Specific timeframes sustain motivation and concentration.

Divide larger goals into smaller milestones: Assign manageable deadlines for each step along the way.

Example (Non-Time-Bound): "Enhance flexibility."

Example (Time-Bound): "Augment hamstring flexibility by 10 degrees within eight weeks."

The SMART Goals methodology is adaptable. Adjust goals as necessary based on progress or evolving circumstances. The essence lies in setting objectives that are specific, measurable, attainable, relevant, and time-bound to optimize success in Parkinson's disease management.

7.2: Implementing SMART Goals for Wellness and Engagement

Despite the challenges posed by Parkinson's disease, you hold the key to steering through them and crafting a rewarding life. This section delves into applying the SMART Goals framework to specific facets of managing Parkinson's disease.

Getting Specific:
Here's how to set SMART goals tailored to different aspects of Parkinson's disease management:

1. Physical Activity:
   - Goal: Enhance strength and flexibility to boost independence in daily tasks.
   - Specific: Engage in biweekly physical therapy sessions for 12 weeks, focusing on core muscle strengthening and upper body flexibility exercises.
   - Measurable: Monitor attendance and progress in exercises such as sit-to-stand repetitions or arm range of motion.

- Attainable: Accessible physical therapy sessions adapted to your schedule and abilities.
- Relevant: Improved strength and flexibility ease daily activities and lessen reliance on assistance.
- Time-bound: Complete the 12-week physical therapy program.

2. Nutrition:
- Goal: Enhance dietary habits for weight management and sustained energy levels.
- Specific: Consult a registered dietitian for a personalized meal plan emphasizing whole foods, fruits, vegetables, and lean proteins.
- Measurable: Track daily calorie intake, weight changes, and energy levels.
- Attainable: Tailored meal plan accommodating preferences and constraints.
- Relevant: Healthy eating boosts energy, reduces fatigue, and enhances overall well-being.
- Time-bound:Schedule a dietitian appointment within a month and adhere to the meal plan for three months.

3. Sleep Hygiene:
- Goal: Improve sleep quality for enhanced daytime vitality.

- Specific: Establish a consistent sleep routine, aiming for 7-8 hours nightly.
- Measurable: Monitor sleep patterns using trackers or journals.
- Attainable: Gradually adjust sleep schedule if needed.
- Relevant: Quality sleep diminishes fatigue and uplifts mood.
- Time-bound: Implement consistent sleep routines for four weeks.

4. Social Connection:
- Goal: Foster social ties to alleviate loneliness.
- Specific: Join a Parkinson's disease support group, attending monthly meetings.
- Measurable: Track attendance and interactions with group members.
- Attainable: Support groups offer understanding and connection.
- Relevant: Social engagement bolsters emotional well-being.
- Time-bound: Commit to group meetings for three months.

These are merely examples; tailor goals to your needs.

Putting Goals into Action:

After setting SMART goals, translate them into action:

1. Action Plan:
   Break goals into manageable steps, identifying needed resources and potential obstacles.
2. Priority:
   Focus on key goals first, adding more later.
3. Support:
   Don't hesitate to seek help from loved ones or professionals.
4. Progress Tracking:
   Regularly monitor progress and celebrate achievements.
5. Flexibility:
   Be ready to adapt goals or plans as circumstances change.

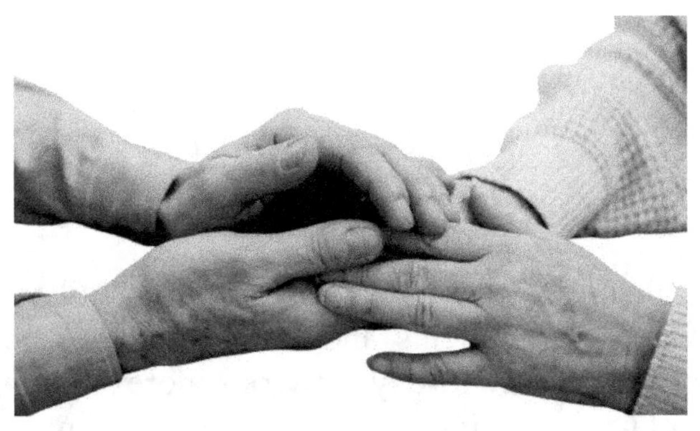

CHAPTER 8: PRACTICAL ADVICE FOR DAILY LIFE

Parkinson's disease may disrupt your daily routine, but with adjustments and smart strategies, you can handle your day-to-day activities more smoothly and maintain your independence longer. This chapter provides practical tips to streamline your daily routine and seize every moment.

Planning and Preparation:

1. Organize Your Day: Kickstart your day by scheduling medications, meals, exercise, and tasks to stay on track and organized.
2. Prep Ahead: Arrange your outfit and gather essentials the night before to avoid morning rushes and stress.
3. Simplify Tasks: Break down complex tasks into smaller steps for easier completion without feeling overwhelmed.
4. Delegate and Seek Help: Don't hesitate to ask for assistance from family, friends, or caregivers to focus your energy on tasks you can manage independently.

Managing Medications:
1. Stick to Schedule: Adhere to your medication regimen as prescribed, using reminders or pill organizers to avoid missing doses.
2. Plan Around Side Effects: Adjust activities to minimize disruptions from medication side effects such as drowsiness.
3. Consult Your Doctor: Discuss any medication-related issues with your doctor for potential adjustments or coping strategies.

Simplifying Daily Activities:
1. Dressing: Opt for comfortable, easy-to-wear clothing with convenient closures like zippers or Velcro.
2. Bathing: Ensure safety with shower chairs or grab bars for added support.
3. Cooking: Prep meals in advance and use utensils with larger handles for better grip.
4. Eating: Cut food into manageable pieces and utilize weighted utensils for improved hand control.

Maintaining Your Home Environment:
1. Declutter: Minimize obstacles by organizing and decluttering your living space.

2. Enhance Lighting: Improve visibility and safety by ensuring adequate lighting throughout your home.
3. Utilize Assistive Devices: Consider grab bars, raised toilet seats, or reachers to enhance accessibility and safety.

Staying Active Throughout the Day:

- Prioritize Exercise: Incorporate exercise into your daily routine to manage Parkinson's symptoms effectively.
- Stay Moving: Find opportunities for physical activity during the day, like taking the stairs or doing stretches.

Prioritizing Rest and Relaxation:

- Listen to Your Body: Schedule rest breaks, especially when feeling fatigued.
- Practice Relaxation: Employ techniques like deep breathing or meditation to manage stress and improve sleep.
- Establish Bedtime Routine: Create a soothing bedtime routine to promote relaxation and better sleep quality.

Staying Socially Connected:

- Schedule Social Time: Make time for social interactions with loved ones or support groups to combat loneliness.

- Utilize Communication Tools: Explore digital tools like video calls to maintain connections, especially if face-to-face interaction is challenging.

Sample Weekly Schedule for a Person with Parkinson's Disease:

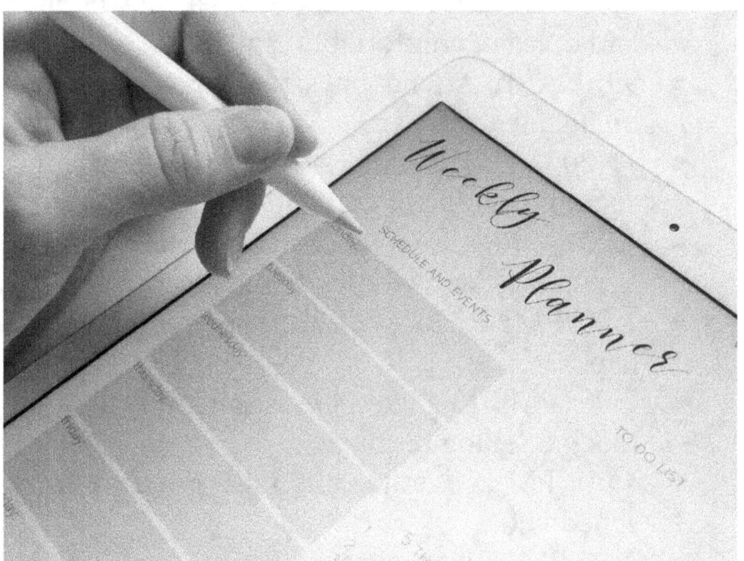

This weekly itinerary illustrates how to integrate practical tips into your daily routine while managing Parkinson's disease. Customize these suggestions to suit your individual needs, preferences, and medication regimen.

Monday:

- 7:00 AM: Wake up, take medication with water, and enjoy a protein and fiber-rich breakfast.
- 7:30 AM: Stretch gently while listening to calming music to enhance flexibility and range of motion.
- 8:00 AM: Shower safely using a shower chair and dress in comfortable clothes.
- 9:00 AM: Attend physical therapy focusing on balance and gait.
- 11:00 AM: Have a healthy snack and socialize online or call a loved one.
- 12:00 PM: Lunch with lean protein, vegetables, and whole grains.
- 1:00 PM: Relax with a book, audiobook, or nap.
- 2:00 PM: Engage in a stimulating activity like gardening or puzzles.
- 4:00 PM: Hydrate and take medication as scheduled.
- 4:30 PM: Take a short walk outdoors.
- 6:00 PM: Enjoy a balanced dinner.
- 7:00 PM: Quality time with loved ones in person or virtually.
- 8:00 PM: Begin a calming bedtime routine with a warm bath.
- 9:00 PM: Take medication and prepare for sleep.

Tuesday:
Similar routine with a support group visit for social interaction and support.

Wednesday:
Replace support group visit with a doctor's appointment for check-up and medication review.

Thursday:
Plan meals and grocery shop for the week, ensuring healthy options.

Friday:
Enjoy a relaxed morning and invite a friend over for social interaction.

Saturday:
Dedicate time to household chores, breaking tasks into manageable steps.

Sunday:
Relax and recharge, engaging in low-key activities and self-care.

Note: Customize the schedule to fit your needs and energy levels, aiming for a balanced and fulfilling lifestyle while managing Parkinson's disease effectively.

8.1: Strategic Meal Planning and Nutrition

Parkinson's disease can affect meal preparation and energy levels, but with strategic meal planning and mindful eating, you can support your body's needs and manage symptoms effectively.

The Significance of Nutrition:

A balanced diet is vital for managing Parkinson's disease as it:

- Boosts Energy: Proper nutrition sustains energy levels, combating fatigue and enabling participation in activities.
- Enhances Mood: Nutrients influence brain function and mood, fostering positivity and emotional well-being.
- Aids Digestion: Dietary fiber promotes gut health, alleviating constipation—a common symptom.
- Optimizes Medication: Meal planning ensures medications are taken optimally, improving absorption.

Creating a Balanced Plate:

Visualize your plate divided into sections for nutritious balance:
1. Half with Veggies: Fill half with non-starchy vegetables for vitamins, minerals, and antioxidants.
2. Quarter with Protein: Allocate a quarter to lean proteins like chicken, fish, or plant-based options.
3. Quarter with Whole Grains: Use the remaining quarter for whole grains for sustained energy and fiber.
4. Incorporate Healthy Fats: Include sources like avocados, nuts, and olive oil for brain health.

Planning and Preparation:

Efficient meal planning streamlines life and ensures healthy options:
- Weekly Meal Plans: Dedicate time weekly to plan meals and make grocery lists.
- Coordinate with Medication: Schedule meals around medication times for optimal absorption.
- Prep Ahead: Cook large batches, portion, and freeze meals for convenience.

- Stock Up on Staples: Maintain a supply of whole grains, beans, and frozen veggies for quick meals.

Further Nutritional Tips:
Consider additional nutritional factors:
- Stay Hydrated: Aim for eight glasses of water daily to support overall health.
- Limit Added Sugars: Reduce intake from processed foods and sugary drinks to manage weight and energy levels.
- Prioritize Fiber: Increase fiber intake for digestion and constipation prevention.
- Consult Professionals: Seek guidance from a dietitian for personalized meal plans.

Facilitating Mealtimes:
Make eating easier and enjoyable with these tips:
1. Opt for Simplicity: Choose straightforward recipes with minimal steps.
2. Use Time-Saving Tools: Employ appliances like slow cookers for efficiency.
3. Seek Assistance: Don't hesitate to ask for help from loved ones or caregivers.
4. Embrace Enjoyment: Create a pleasant dining atmosphere to savor meals with others.

7-Day Meal Plan for Parkinson's Disease Management

This evidence-based meal plan spans 7 days, designed to support individuals with Parkinson's disease by prioritizing balanced nutrition, addressing tremors and medication interactions, and simplifying meal prep.

General Considerations:
- Embrace Whole Foods: Prioritize unprocessed foods like fruits, veggies, whole grains, lean proteins, and healthy fats.
- Balanced Meals: Each meal should feature protein, complex carbs, and healthy fats for sustained energy and nutrient absorption.
- Stay Hydrated: Aim for eight glasses of water daily to support overall health and medication effectiveness.
- Control Portions: Listen to hunger cues, and opt for smaller plates to manage portion sizes effectively.
- Medication Awareness: Consult your doctor about potential medication-food interactions, especially regarding levodopa absorption.

Sample 7-Day Meal Plan:

Day 1 (Monday):
- Breakfast: Greek yogurt with berries and granola for a mix of protein, fiber, and probiotics.
- Mid-Morning Snack: Apple slices with almond butter for fiber and healthy fats.
- Lunch: Leftover grilled chicken with brown rice and roasted veggies for balanced nutrition.
- Afternoon Snack: Mixed nuts and dried cranberries for a satisfying, nutrient-packed snack.
- Dinner: Baked salmon with sweet potato and broccoli for lean protein and essential vitamins.

Day 2 (Tuesday):
- Breakfast: Scrambled eggs with whole-wheat toast and avocado for protein and healthy fats.
- Mid-Morning Snack: Cottage cheese with cucumber and tomato slices for protein and hydration.
- Lunch: Lentil soup with whole-wheat roll and side salad for plant-based protein and fiber.
- Afternoon Snack: Banana with peanut butter for quick energy and healthy fats.
- Dinner: Turkey chili with whole-wheat crackers for protein and fiber.

Days 3-7 (Wednesday-Sunday):
These days offer diverse meal options while maintaining nutrition and ease of preparation. Adapt based on personal preferences and dietary needs.

Additional Tips:

Streamline Prep: Use time-saving tools like slow cookers and prep meals in advance.
Tremor Management: Opt for utensils with thicker handles and weighted options for easier handling.
Socialize: Enjoy meals with loved ones for a more enjoyable dining experience.

This plan is a guide. Consult a dietitian for personalized advice to effectively manage Parkinson's disease and enjoy a fulfilling life.

8.2: Streamlining Household Tasks and Daily Routines

Parkinson's disease can pose challenges with daily tasks, but with strategic adjustments and practical tools, you can simplify routines and preserve independence.

- Task Breakdown: Divide large tasks into smaller steps for easier completion and reduced overwhelm.
- Scheduled Chores: Create a routine schedule for household tasks to ensure they're accomplished without stress.
- List Keeping: Use to-do lists to track chores and errands, boosting motivation and task completion.

Optimizing Your Environment:

Decluttering: Minimize clutter to enhance safety and reduce stress, allocating items to designated storage or donating unused belongings.

Lighting Enhancement: Improve visibility with adequate lighting, especially in high-traffic areas like bathrooms and kitchens.

Assistive Tools: Utilize grab bars, raised seats, or reachers for increased safety and accessibility.

Simplifying Daily Tasks:

1. Meal Prep: Freeze pre-made meals for convenience, and opt for kitchen tools with ergonomic handles.
2. Cleaning: Tackle one area at a time using user-friendly cleaning products, and consider delegating tasks or hiring help.

3. Laundry: Wash smaller loads and use wheeled baskets for easier handling.
4. Dressing: Choose clothing with simple closures and lay out outfits in advance.

Energy Management:

- Pacing: Pace yourself throughout the day to manage fatigue, scheduling rest breaks as needed.
- Task Prioritization: Focus on essential tasks first to ensure completion, adjusting based on energy levels.

Safety Measures:

- Non-Slip Surfaces: Install non-slip mats in wet areas like bathrooms to prevent falls.
- Rug Security: Secure loose rugs to prevent tripping hazards.
- Clear Pathways: Keep walkways clutter-free for safe navigation.

Seeking Assistance:

Accepting Help: Don't hesitate to enlist support from loved ones or home care services to conserve energy and maintain independence.

CHAPTER 9: FAMILY AND CAREGIVER ASSISTANCE

Parkinson's disease affects not only the diagnosed individual but also their loved ones. Family members play a vital role in offering emotional support, aiding with daily activities, and advocating for their well-being. This chapter delves into the significance of family support and provides tools for effectively navigating this journey.

9.1: Assistance for Family Members

A diagnosis of Parkinson's disease can overwhelm both the diagnosed person and their family. Here's how you, as a family member, can provide support and navigate this journey with resilience and empathy:

1. Educate Yourself:
Understand Parkinson's: Knowledge empowers. Educate yourself about the disease, its symptoms, and progression to comprehend your loved one's challenges and make informed decisions about their care.

Trustworthy Sources: Seek information from credible sources like the Parkinson's Foundation or the National Institute on Neurological Disorders and Stroke.

2. Effective Communication:

Open Dialogue: Foster open and honest communication with your loved one. Address their concerns, fears, and needs while providing a safe space for expression.

Listening: Practice active listening without judgment, offering empathy and support to your loved one.

Collaborate with Caregivers: Maintain clear communication with healthcare professionals involved in your loved one's care to ensure a cohesive care plan.

3. Emotional Support:

Patience and Understanding: Understand the emotional changes Parkinson's can induce and offer patience and understanding.

Validate Feelings: Acknowledge and validate your loved one's feelings, offering unwavering support and understanding.

Maintain Positivity: Focus on the positives, celebrating achievements and finding moments of joy amidst challenges.

4. Practical Assistance:

Aid with Daily Activities:
As the disease progresses, assist with daily tasks such as bathing, dressing, and meal preparation, enabling independence.

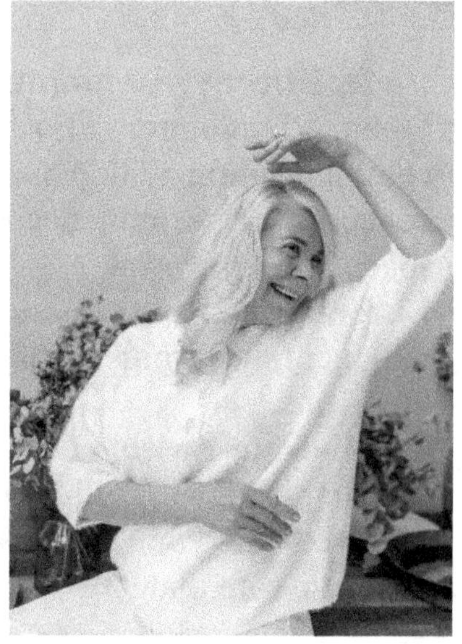

Manage Appointments and Medications: Help with scheduling appointments, medication management, and treatment plans to ease the burden.

Provide Transportation: Offer transportation for appointments and errands if driving becomes challenging, ensuring connectivity and normalcy.

5. Self-Care:

Prioritize Your Well-being: Caregiving can be taxing, so prioritize self-care activities to manage stress and well-being.

Seek Support: Join caregiver support groups, talk to a therapist, or confide in trusted individuals to cope with challenges effectively.

Maintain Healthy Habits: Attend to your physical and mental health by maintaining a balanced lifestyle with proper nutrition, exercise, and sufficient rest. This ensures you can provide stronger support to your loved one.

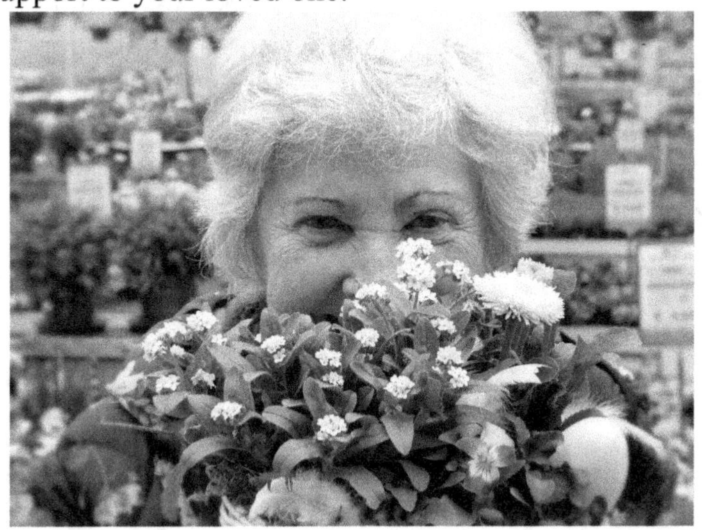

CHAPTER 10: GAZING AHEAD

Parkinson's disease progresses, yet your future isn't devoid of hope. By planning ahead, maintaining a positive mindset, and relying on familial support, you can navigate the journey ahead and continue leading a gratifying life. This chapter delves into strategies for preparing for the future and adapting to forthcoming changes.

10.1: Strategic Future Planning with Parkinson's Disease

A Parkinson's diagnosis may instigate apprehension about what lies ahead. Nonetheless, strategic planning empowers you to seize control and make informed decisions. Here are key considerations:

1. Financial Preparation:
   Collaborate with a trusted financial advisor to plan for potential healthcare expenses and long-term care needs. Update legal documents like wills and power of attorney for clarity.
2. Advance Directives:

Establish directives outlining medical preferences for instances when you're unable to communicate, ensuring your values guide decision-making.

3. Legal Affairs:
   Seek guidance from an elder law attorney to address legal matters such as guardianship and estate planning, securing your affairs and honoring your desires.

4. Long-Term Care Exploration:
   Research various long-term care options and discuss preferences with family to establish a plan aligned with your needs.

5. Open Communication:
   Foster transparent discussions with loved ones about future requirements and preferences to ensure readiness for evolving circumstances.

6. Research Engagement:
   Stay informed about Parkinson's research and advocacy, potentially participating in trials or studies to advance treatment development.

Assembling Your Support Team:

Doctor-Patient Relationship: Cultivate a strong bond with your neurologist, maintaining candid communication about symptoms and treatment objectives.

Specialist Consultations:

Consider consultations with specialists like physical therapists, occupational therapists, or mental health professionals to address specific needs.

Caregiver Network:

Identify reliable individuals for support with daily tasks and consider professional caregiver services if necessary.

Social Support:

Engage with Parkinson's support groups for mutual learning, sharing experiences, and building a supportive community.

Preparing for the future may feel daunting, but take it step by step. Begin by gathering information, conferring with loved ones, and assembling a robust care network to accompany you on your journey.

10.2: Embracing Change and Embracing the Unknown

Parkinson's is progressive, and change is inevitable. Here's how to adapt and manage uncertainty:

- Focus on Controllables:

Direct energy towards what you can control, such as daily routines, exercise, and stress management, fostering resilience in the face of change.

- Embrace Adaptability:

Stay open to adjusting routines and activities as needs evolve, embracing new approaches to symptom management.

- Cultivate Coping Strategies:

Develop healthy coping mechanisms to navigate stress and anxiety, integrating practices like deep breathing or mindfulness.

- Present-Centric Living:

Reduce future-related anxiety by living in the present, cherishing relationships and finding joy in everyday moments.

- Positivity Cultivation:

Maintain an optimistic outlook, celebrating small victories and looking towards future possibilities.

- Accept Assistance:

Don't hesitate to seek support from loved ones or professionals, as accepting help prolongs independence.

- Professional Guidance:

Consider counseling or therapy for support in managing emotional challenges and adapting to change effectively.

CONCLUSION

This book has provided you with a plethora of information and practical strategies to navigate your Parkinson's disease journey. Remember, you're not alone in this endeavor. Countless individuals worldwide are leading fulfilling lives despite Parkinson's, and you too can overcome challenges and embrace opportunities.

We recognize that a Parkinson's diagnosis can be daunting. However, as you've delved into these chapters, you've uncovered a roadmap for managing your daily life, addressing symptoms, and prioritizing your health. We've stressed the significance of a balanced diet, regular physical activity, and a supportive community – all essential elements for thriving with Parkinson's.

Empowering Knowledge and Action
Knowledge empowers action. Armed with information about Parkinson's, its symptoms, and treatment options, you can actively engage in your healthcare decisions. Don't hesitate to ask questions, express concerns, and collaborate with your healthcare team.

Embracing Change, Embracing Life
While Parkinson's may introduce changes, it doesn't diminish your capacity for happiness and

fulfillment. Focus on what you can control – your mindset, routines, and symptom management approach. Celebrate every achievement, remain receptive to new opportunities, and tackle the journey with bravery and resilience.

Thank you for choosing this book as your companion. We believe in your inner strength, resilience, and ability to lead a vibrant life despite Parkinson's. Remember, the resources and support networks outlined in this book are within reach. Take advantage of them, connect with your community, and empower yourself to thrive, not just survive, with Parkinson's.

Wishing you all the best on your journey. May it be filled with resilience, optimism, and moments of joy and connection.

ISBN 9798320672793

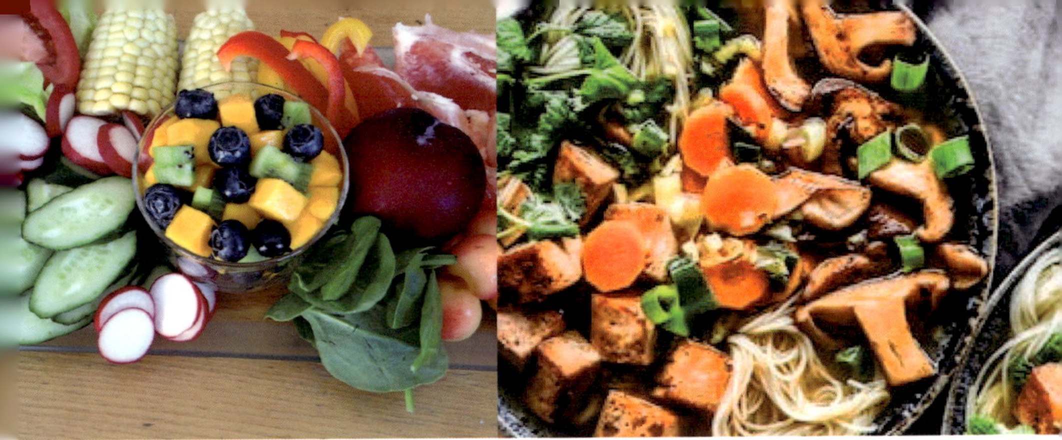

HE ULTIMATE
PLANT BASED GUT HEALTH COOKBOOK

our Essential Cookbook for Easy and Delicious Plant-Based Recipes for a Healthy Gut and Digestive Health.

IRISTIANA WHITE

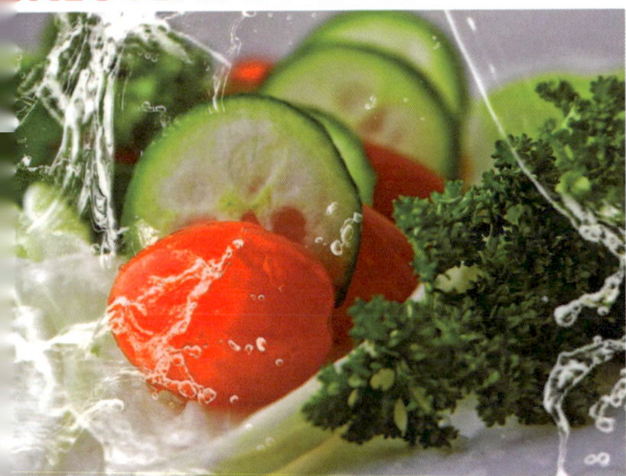

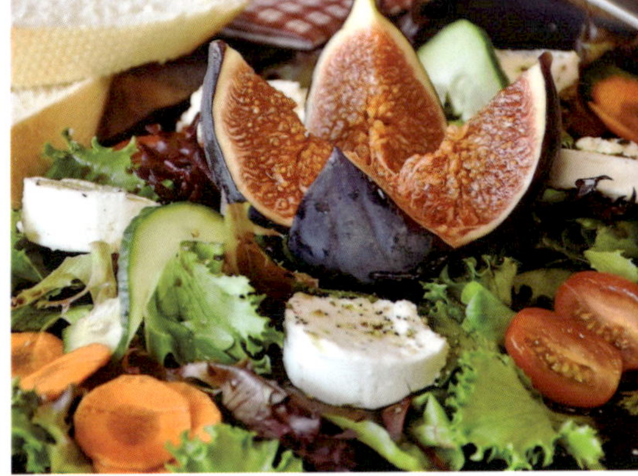

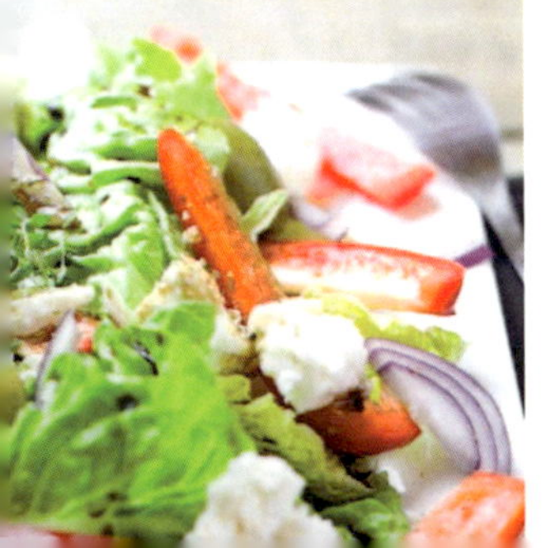

BONUS

14-DAY MEAL PLAN

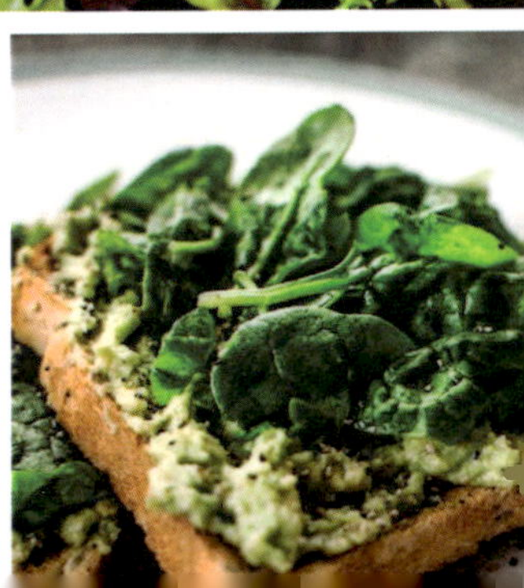